Using Your Journal

Hey girl! I'm so excited you have this journal in your hands right now!

There are probably two circumstances in which you found this journal:

1.) A fellow mama gifted it to you, or 2.) You picked up this journal yourself to help you through this whole new mommy thing.

If you received this journal as a gift from a fellow mama, give her a smooch. She loves you and cares about YOUR well being during this new season of life you're in. If you purchased this journal for yourself, girl, you are ahead of the game! Way to acknowledge your need for some self-care and love. I'm proud of you.

In this journal you will find simple, yet profound ways to care for yourself during this season of life. So often as mamas we put ourselves last. It is critical that we take care of ourselves. This comes in the form of our physical health like nutrition and personal hygiene, to our mental and emotional health in the form of communicating our needs and filling our own cups.

One of the most beneficial aspects to purchasing this journal is that it gives you exclusive access to our online community! Please join us by requesting to join the "Mama Matters, Too" Facebook group. You will be given access within 24 hours of your request!

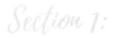

- **Mommy Mantra:** This is a short, positive, mommy quote that will start your day off with a little empowerment, gut check, or giggle.
- **Today I Am Grateful For:** Pair a statement of gratitude with your mommy mantra and you are starting your day of mentally STRONG!
- **Got Dressed And Ready For The Day:** Keep it simple. This can mean a 15 minute shower, leggings, and a swipe of mascara.
- **Food/Water/Exercise:** As a mama, we often forget to fuel our own bodies! Filling our tanks with healthy foods, lots of water, and engaging in daily physical activity does wonders for the mind, body, and soul.

Section 2:

- **Mommy Time:** Having 30 minutes to yourself every single day will allow you to feel like "you" again. This can be a shower, walk, time to read, or sitting in the parking lot of a coffee shop with a latte!
- **Personal/Spiritual Development:** Investing in your personal development and/or spiritual development will empower and equip you for life's trials. This can be in the form of a devotional, book, or audio book.
- **Went Outside:** Even if it's raining, step outside. Breathe the fresh air. It can truly rejuvenate you and give you a bit of new found energy.
- **Connected with Spouse:** This can be very hard when you are a new mom. Connecting with your spouse can simply be 10 minutes of coffee talk on the couch at the end of the day, going for a walk together, reading a couples' devotional each morning, or sharing your highlight of the day over dinner and discussing it.
- **Talked to a Friend:** Remember to reach out to a friend each day to avoid isolation. Participating in mommy and me classes as well as engaging in our online Facebook group will give you a sense of community and belonging.
- **Asked for Help:** Whether being a mommy is a breeze for you, or you are deep in the throes of postpartum depression, we all need a little help sometimes.

If you think you may be struggling with a mental health disorder, I urge you to seek the counsel of your OB on how to navigate this season. Do not waste time. You can live a better quality of life. Permit yourself to do that.

Feelings/Sweet Moments/Other Notes: Use this section to reflect on your feelings that day, some special moments you want to record, and anything else you want to remember.

Weekly Reflection: At the end of each week you will see a page for reflection. Take the time to use this page as a tool to better the quality of your daily life as a mama.

Always remember that your goal isn't to be perfect, mama. It's to take care of yourself and that baby. If you don't knock it out of the park some days, that's OKAY, and to be expected! Grace, sweet girl, grace.

My hope is that this journal gives you the permission and intentionality in taking time for yourself each day, in simple yet profound ways. Being a mama is the most beautiful blessing, yet can be the most difficult and trying aspect of our lives. Allow this journal to guide you toward healthy balance in your life.

You are not alone.
You are the exact mama that your babies need.
You are doing a great job.

*Love Your Fellow Mama
In The Trenches,*

Lyss

Monday

I still remember the days I prayed for the things I have now. –Unknown

I am Grateful For:

breakfast   lunch   dinner   snacks   exercise

got dressed and ready for the day

30 min. mommy time	personal/spiritual development	went outside
connected with spouse	talked to a friend	asked for help

Feelings, sweet moments, and other notes:

Tuesday

Bad moments don't make bad moms.
-Lysa Terkeurst

I am
Grateful
For:

breakfast   lunch   dinner   snacks   exercise

got dressed and ready for the day

| 30 min. mommy time | personal/spiritual development | went outside |
| connected with spouse | talked to a friend | asked for help |

Feelings, sweet moments, and other notes:

Wednesday

There is no way to be a perfect mother, but a million ways to be a great one. –Jill Churchill

I am Grateful For:

breakfast   lunch   dinner   snacks   exercise

~~~~~~~~~~~~~~~~~~~~~~~~~~~~~~~

got dressed and ready for the day

| 30 min. mommy time | personal/spiritual development | went outside |

| connected with spouse | talked to a friend | asked for help |

Feelings, sweet moments, and other notes:

Thursday

Successful mothers are not the ones that have never struggled, they are the ones that never gave up, despite their struggles. –Sharon Jaynes

I am Grateful For:

breakfast   lunch   dinner   snacks   exercise

got dressed and ready for the day

30 min. mommy time	personal/spiritual development	went outside
connected with spouse	talked to a friend	asked for help

Feelings, sweet moments, and other notes:

Friday

Life is tough, my darling, but so are you.
-Stephanie Bennett-Henry

I am Grateful For:

breakfast   lunch   dinner   snacks   exercise

~~~~~~~~~~~~~~~~~~~~~~~~~~~~~

got dressed and ready for the day

30 min. mommy time	personal/spiritual development	went outside
connected with spouse	talked to a friend	asked for help

Feelings, sweet moments, and other notes:

Saturday

This mothering role will teach you more about yourself than you ever expected. –Tricia Goyer

I am Grateful For:

breakfast   lunch   dinner   snacks   exercise

~~~~~~~~~~~~~~~~~~~~~~~~~~~~~~~~~~

got dressed and ready for the day

| 30 min. mommy time | personal/spiritual development | went outside |
| connected with spouse | talked to a friend | asked for help |

Feelings, sweet moments, and other notes:

Sunday

Giving grace to yourself is never more important than when you become a mother. –Whitney Meade

I am Grateful For:

breakfast   lunch   dinner   snacks   exercise

⌣⌣⌣⌣⌣⌣⌣⌣⌣⌣⌣⌣⌣⌣⌣

got dressed and ready for the day

30 min. mommy time	personal/spiritual development	went outside
connected with spouse	talked to a friend	asked for help

Feelings, sweet moments, and other notes:

Weekly Reflection

My greatest struggle this week was...

I'm proud of myself this week because...

Next week I want to focus on....

I am a great mama.

Monday

Don't be afraid to speak up for yourself. Keep fighting for your dreams! ~ Gabby Douglas

I am Grateful For:

breakfast　　lunch　　dinner　　snacks　　exercise

~~~~~~~~~~~~~~~~~~~~~~~~~~~~~~~

got dressed and ready for the day

30 min. mommy time	personal/spiritual development	went outside
connected with spouse	talked to a friend	asked for help

Feelings, sweet moments, and other notes:

Tuesday

I'm where I'm meant to be.
-Rapunzel, Tangled

I am Grateful For:

breakfast   lunch   dinner   snacks   exercise

~~~~~~~~~~~~~~~~~~~~~~~~~~~~

got dressed and ready for the day

| 30 min. mommy time | personal/spiritual development | went outside |
| connected with spouse | talked to a friend | asked for help |

Feelings, sweet moments, and other notes:

Wednesday

You can't experience simple joys when you're living life with your hair on fire. –Emily Ley

I am Grateful For:

breakfast   lunch   dinner   snacks   exercise

~~~~~~~~~~~~~~~~~~~~~~~

got dressed and ready for the day

| 30 min. mommy time | personal/spiritual development | went outside |
| connected with spouse | talked to a friend | asked for help |

Feelings, sweet moments, and other notes:

Thursday

A baby fills a place in your heart you never knew was empty. –Unknown

I am Grateful For:

breakfast   lunch   dinner   snacks   exercise

got dressed and ready for the day

30 min. mommy time	personal/spiritual development	went outside
connected with spouse	talked to a friend	asked for help

Feelings, sweet moments, and other notes:

Friday

If you can't find beauty in the ugliness, you won't find it in the beauty either. —Joanna Gaines

I am Grateful For:

breakfast   lunch   dinner   snacks   exercise

~~~~~~~~~~~~~~~~~~~~~~~~~

got dressed and ready for the day

| 30 min. mommy time | personal/spiritual development | went outside |
| connected with spouse | talked to a friend | asked for help |

Feelings, sweet moments, and other notes:

Saturday

She opens her mouth in wisdom and the teaching of kindness is upon her tongue. Proverbs 31:26

I am Grateful For:

breakfast   lunch   dinner   snacks   exercise

got dressed and ready for the day

30 min. mommy time	personal/spiritual development	went outside
connected with spouse	talked to a friend	asked for help

Feelings, sweet moments, and other notes:

Sunday

Our words have power, but our actions shape lives.
–Rachel Hollis

I am
Grateful
For:

breakfast   lunch   dinner   snacks   exercise

got dressed and ready for the day

30 min. mommy time	personal/spiritual development	went outside
connected with spouse	talked to a friend	asked for help

Feelings, sweet moments, and other notes:

Weekly Reflection

My greatest struggle this week was...

I'm proud of myself this week because...

Next week I want to focus on....

I am a great mama.

Monday

Today's special moments are tomorrow's memories.
–Genie, The Return of Jafar

I am Grateful For:

breakfast   lunch   dinner   snacks   exercise

~~~~~~~~~~~~~~~~~~~~~~~~~~~~~~~~~~~~~~~

got dressed and ready for the day

30 min. mommy time	personal/spiritual development	went outside
connected with spouse	talked to a friend	asked for help

Feelings, sweet moments, and other notes:

Tuesday

If you're a mom, you're a superhero, period.
- Rosie Pope

I am Grateful For:

breakfast   lunch   dinner   snacks   exercise

~~~~~~~~~~~~~~~~~~~~

got dressed and ready for the day

| 30 min. mommy time | personal/spiritual development | went outside |
| connected with spouse | talked to a friend | asked for help |

Feelings, sweet moments, and other notes:

Wednesday

Don't let today's reaction become tomorrow's regret.
– Lysa Terkeurst

I am Grateful For:

breakfast   lunch   dinner   snacks   exercise

~~~~~~~~~~~~~~~~~~~~~~

got dressed and ready for the day

30 min. mommy time	personal/spiritual development	went outside
connected with spouse	talked to a friend	asked for help

Feelings, sweet moments, and other notes:

Thursday

Sometimes the smallest step in the right direction ends up being the biggest step of your life. -Emily Ley

I am Grateful For:

breakfast   lunch   dinner   snacks   exercise

∿∿∿∿∿∿∿∿∿∿∿∿

got dressed and ready for the day

30 min. mommy time	personal/spiritual development	went outside
connected with spouse	talked to a friend	asked for help

Feelings, sweet moments, and other notes:

Friday

Sometimes the littlest things take up the biggest room in your heart. —Winnie The Pooh

I am Grateful For:

breakfast   lunch   dinner   snacks   exercise

~~~~~~~~~~~~~~~~~~~~~~~~~~

got dressed and ready for the day

| 30 min. mommy time | personal/spiritual development | went outside |
| connected with spouse | talked to a friend | asked for help |

Feelings, sweet moments, and other notes:

Saturday

We can all choose to be atmosphere changers.
—Joanna Gaines

I am
Grateful
For:

breakfast   lunch   dinner   snacks   exercise

got dressed and ready for the day

30 min. mommy time	personal/spiritual development	went outside
connected with spouse	talked to a friend	asked for help

Feelings, sweet moments, and other notes:

Sunday

Even miracles take a little time.
– Fairy Godmother, Cinderella

I am Grateful For:

breakfast   lunch   dinner   snacks   exercise

~~~~~~~~~~~~~~~~~~~~~~~~~~~~

got dressed and ready for the day

| 30 min. mommy time | personal/spiritual development | went outside |
| connected with spouse | talked to a friend | asked for help |

Feelings, sweet moments, and other notes:

Weekly Reflection

My greatest struggle this week was...

I'm proud of myself this week because...

Next week I want to focus on....

I am a great mama.

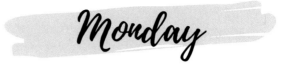

Monday

I've often called mothers the greatest spiritual teachers in the world. –Oprah

I am Grateful For:

breakfast   lunch   dinner   snacks   exercise

got dressed and ready for the day

30 min. mommy time	personal/spiritual development	went outside
connected with spouse	talked to a friend	asked for help

Feelings, sweet moments, and other notes:

Tuesday

Motherhood is a million little moments that God weaves together with grace, redemption, laughter, tears, and most of all, love.
-Lysa Terkeurst

I am Grateful For:

breakfast   lunch   dinner   snacks   exercise

∿∿∿∿∿∿∿∿∿∿∿∿∿∿

got dressed and ready for the day

30 min. mommy time	personal/spiritual development	went outside
connected with spouse	talked to a friend	asked for help

Feelings, sweet moments, and other notes:

Wednesday

Your influence as a mother is powerful. Don't waste it.
Little eyes are watching you. –Unknown

I am Grateful For:

breakfast   lunch   dinner   snacks   exercise

got dressed and ready for the day

30 min. mommy time	personal/spiritual development	went outside
connected with spouse	talked to a friend	asked for help

Feelings, sweet moments, and other notes:

Thursday

Remember, you're the one who can fill the world with sunshine.
—Snow White, Snow White and the Seven Dwarfs

I am Grateful For:

breakfast   lunch   dinner   snacks   exercise

got dressed and ready for the day

| 30 min. mommy time | personal/spiritual development | went outside |
| connected with spouse | talked to a friend | asked for help |

Feelings, sweet moments, and other notes:

Friday

The very fact that you worry about being a good mom means that you are one. —Jodi Picoult

I am Grateful For:

breakfast   lunch   dinner   snacks   exercise

~~~~~~~~~~~~~~~~~~~~~~~~~~~~~

got dressed and ready for the day

| 30 min. mommy time | personal/spiritual development | went outside |
| connected with spouse | talked to a friend | asked for help |

Feelings, sweet moments, and other notes:

Saturday

When life is sweet say thank you and celebrate. When life is bitter say thank you and grow. – Shauna Niequist

I am
Grateful
For:

breakfast   lunch   dinner   snacks   exercise

got dressed and ready for the day

| 30 min. mommy time | personal/spiritual development | went outside |
| connected with spouse | talked to a friend | asked for help |

Feelings, sweet moments, and other notes:

Sunday

There will be so many times you feel like you failed. But in the eyes, ears, and mind of your child, you are a super mom. –Stephanie Precourt

I am Grateful For:

breakfast   lunch   dinner   snacks   exercise

~~~~~~~~~~~~~~~~~~~~~~~~~~~~~~~~~~~~~

got dressed and ready for the day

| 30 min. mommy time | personal/spiritual development | went outside |
| connected with spouse | talked to a friend | asked for help |

Feelings, sweet moments, and other notes:

Weekly Reflection

My greatest struggle this week was...

I'm proud of myself this week because...

Next week I want to focus on....

I am a great mama.

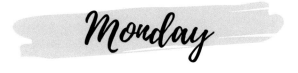

Monday

Interrupt anxiety with gratitude. –Rachel Hollis

I am Grateful For:

breakfast   lunch   dinner   snacks   exercise

~~~~~~~~~~~~~~~~~~~~~~~~~~~~~~~~~

got dressed and ready for the day

30 min. mommy time	personal/spiritual development	went outside
connected with spouse	talked to a friend	asked for help

Feelings, sweet moments, and other notes:

Tuesday

I will hold myself to a standard of grace, not perfection.
-Emily Ley

I am
Grateful
For:

breakfast   lunch   dinner   snacks   exercise

〜〜〜〜〜〜〜〜〜〜〜〜〜〜〜

got dressed and ready for the day

30 min. mommy time	personal/spiritual development	went outside
connected with spouse	talked to a friend	asked for help

Feelings, sweet moments, and other notes:

Wednesday

There is an abundant need in this world for your exact brand of beautiful. -Lysa Terkeurst

I am Grateful For:

breakfast   lunch   dinner   snacks   exercise

~~~~~~~~~~~~~~~~~~~~~~~~~~~~

got dressed and ready for the day

30 min. mommy time	personal/spiritual development	went outside
connected with spouse	talked to a friend	asked for help

Feelings, sweet moments, and other notes:

Thursday

My mother...she is softened at the edges and tempered with a spine of steel. I want to grow old and be like her. –Jodi Picoult

I am Grateful For:

breakfast   lunch   dinner   snacks   exercise

got dressed and ready for the day

30 min. mommy time	personal/spiritual development	went outside
connected with spouse	talked to a friend	asked for help

Feelings, sweet moments, and other notes:

Friday

It never hurts to keep looking for sunshine.
-Eeyore, Winnie the Pooh

I am Grateful For:

breakfast   lunch   dinner   snacks   exercise

~~~~~~~~~~~~~~~~~~~~~~~~~~~~~~~~~~~~~

got dressed and ready for the day

30 min. mommy time	personal/spiritual development	went outside
connected with spouse	talked to a friend	asked for help

Feelings, sweet moments, and other notes:

Saturday

No one's really doing it perfectly, I just think you love your kids with your whole heart, and you do the best you possibly can.
—Reese Witherspoon

I am Grateful For:

breakfast   lunch   dinner   snacks   exercise

~~~~~~~~~~~~~~~~~~~~~~~~~~~~~~

got dressed and ready for the day

| 30 min. mommy time | personal/spiritual development | went outside |
| connected with spouse | talked to a friend | asked for help |

Feelings, sweet moments, and other notes:

Sunday

She is clothed in strength and dignity and laughs without fear of the future. Proverbs 31:25

I am Grateful For:

breakfast   lunch   dinner   snacks   exercise

〰〰〰〰〰〰〰〰〰〰〰

got dressed and ready for the day

| 30 min. mommy time | personal/spiritual development | went outside |
| connected with spouse | talked to a friend | asked for help |

Feelings, sweet moments, and other notes:

Weekly Reflection

My greatest struggle this week was...

I'm proud of myself this week because...

Next week I want to focus on....

I am a great mama.

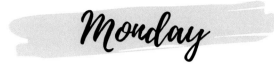

Monday

You don't have to do it all by yourself.
-Elizabeth Dehn

I am Grateful For:

breakfast   lunch   dinner   snacks   exercise

got dressed and ready for the day

| 30 min. mommy time | personal/spiritual development | went outside |
| connected with spouse | talked to a friend | asked for help |

Feelings, sweet moments, and other notes:

Tuesday

It's okay to make mistakes and it's okay to not be good at everything. -Unknown

I am Grateful For:

breakfast   lunch   dinner   snacks   exercise

got dressed and ready for the day

30 min. mommy time	personal/spiritual development	went outside
connected with spouse	talked to a friend	asked for help

Feelings, sweet moments, and other notes:

Wednesday

Sleep at this point is just a concept, something I'm looking forward to investigating in the future. –Amy Poehler

I am Grateful For:

breakfast   lunch   dinner   snacks   exercise

~~~~~~~~~~~~~~~~~~~~~~~~~~~~~~~~~

got dressed and ready for the day

| 30 min. mommy time | personal/spiritual development | went outside |

| connected with spouse | talked to a friend | asked for help |

Feelings, sweet moments, and other notes:

Thursday

You're better than you believe, stronger than you seem, and smarter than you think.

—Christopher Robins, Winnie the Pooh

I am Grateful For:

breakfast   lunch   dinner   snacks   exercise

~~~~~~~~~~~~~~~~~~

got dressed and ready for the day

30 min. mommy time	personal/spiritual development	went outside
connected with spouse	talked to a friend	asked for help

Feelings, sweet moments, and other notes:

Friday

One day you will look back and see that all along, you were blooming. —Morgan Harper Nichols

I am Grateful For:

breakfast   lunch   dinner   snacks   exercise

~~~~~~~~~~~~~~~~~~~~~~~~~~~~~~~~~~

got dressed and ready for the day

30 min. mommy time	personal/spiritual development	went outside
connected with spouse	talked to a friend	asked for help

Feelings, sweet moments, and other notes:

Saturday

Beauty begins the moment you decide to be yourself.
–Coco Chanel

I am Grateful For:

breakfast   lunch   dinner   snacks   exercise

~~~~~~

got dressed and ready for the day

| 30 min. mommy time | personal/spiritual development | went outside |
| connected with spouse | talked to a friend | asked for help |

Feelings, sweet moments, and other notes:

Sunday

I do know one thing about me: I don't measure myself by others' expectations or let others define my worth.
— Sonia Sotomayo

I am Grateful For:

breakfast   lunch   dinner   snacks   exercise

got dressed and ready for the day

30 min. mommy time	personal/spiritual development	went outside
connected with spouse	talked to a friend	asked for help

Feelings, sweet moments, and other notes:

Weekly Reflection

My greatest struggle this week was...

I'm proud of myself this week because...

Next week I want to focus on....

I am a great mama.

Monday

Above all, be the heroine of your life, not the victim.
— Nora Ephron

I am Grateful For:

breakfast   lunch   dinner   snacks   exercise

~~~~~~

got dressed and ready for the day

30 min. mommy time	personal/spiritual development	went outside
connected with spouse	talked to a friend	asked for help

Feelings, sweet moments, and other notes:

Tuesday

I've learned something about kids — they don't do what you say; they do what you do. -Jennifer Lopez

I am Grateful For:

breakfast   lunch   dinner   snacks   exercise

~~~~~~~~~~~~~~~~~~~~~~~~~

got dressed and ready for the day

30 min. mommy time	personal/spiritual development	went outside
connected with spouse	talked to a friend	asked for help

Feelings, sweet moments, and other notes:

Wednesday

I'm not afraid of storms, for I'm learning to sail my ship.
— Louisa May Alcott

I am
Grateful
For:

breakfast   lunch   dinner   snacks   exercise

~~~~~~~~~~~~~~~~~~~~~~~~~~~~~~~~

got dressed and ready for the day

30 min. mommy time	personal/spiritual development	went outside
connected with spouse	talked to a friend	asked for help

Feelings, sweet moments, and other notes:

Thursday

I know for sure that what we dwell on is what we become.
— Oprah Winfrey

I am Grateful For:

breakfast   lunch   dinner   snacks   exercise

~~~~~~~~~~~~~~~~~~~~

got dressed and ready for the day

30 min. mommy time	personal/spiritual development	went outside
connected with spouse	talked to a friend	asked for help

Feelings, sweet moments, and other notes:

Friday

While we try to teach our children about life, our children teach us what life is all about. —Angela Schwindt

I am Grateful For:

breakfast   lunch   dinner   snacks   exercise

~~~~~~~~~~~~~~~~~~~~~~

got dressed and ready for the day

30 min.   personal/spiritual   went
mommy time   development   outside

connected   talked to   asked
with spouse   a friend   for help

Feelings, sweet moments, and other notes:

Saturday

Giving grace to yourself is never more important than when you become a mother. –Whitney Meade

I am Grateful For:

breakfast   lunch   dinner   snacks   exercise

got dressed and ready for the day

30 min.
mommy time

personal/spiritual
development

went
outside

connected
with spouse

talked to
a friend

asked
for help

Feelings, sweet moments, and other notes:

Sunday

Being a mom has made me so tired. And so happy.
— Tina Fey

I am Grateful For:

breakfast   lunch   dinner   snacks   exercise

~~~~~~~~~~~~~~~~~~~~~~

got dressed and ready for the day

| 30 min. mommy time | personal/spiritual development | went outside |
| connected with spouse | talked to a friend | asked for help |

Feelings, sweet moments, and other notes:

Weekly Reflection

My greatest struggle this week was...

I'm proud of myself this week because...

Next week I want to focus on....

I am a great mama.

Monday

I don't have to chase extraordinary moments to find happiness — it's right in front of me if I'm paying attention and practicing gratitude."
- Brené Brown

I am Grateful For:

breakfast   lunch   dinner   snacks   exercise

~~~~~~~~~~~~~~~~~~~~~~~~~

got dressed and ready for the day

30 min. mommy time	personal/spiritual development	went outside
connected with spouse	talked to a friend	asked for help

Feelings, sweet moments, and other notes:

Tuesday

So now faith, hope, and love abide, these three; but the greatest of these is love. 1 Corinthians 13:13

I am Grateful For:

breakfast   lunch   dinner   snacks   exercise

~~~~~~~~~~~~~~~~~~~~~~~~~~~~

got dressed and ready for the day

30 min. mommy time	personal/spiritual development	went outside
connected with spouse	talked to a friend	asked for help

Feelings, sweet moments, and other notes:

Wednesday

I've never had more appreciation for anyone in my entire life until I became a mom. – Chrissy Teigen

I am Grateful For:

breakfast   lunch   dinner   snacks   exercise

~~~~~~~~~~~~~~~~~~~~~~~

got dressed and ready for the day

30 min. mommy time	personal/spiritual development	went outside
connected with spouse	talked to a friend	asked for help

Feelings, sweet moments, and other notes:

Thursday

The fastest way to break the cycle of perfectionism and become a fearless mother is to give up the idea of doing it perfectly — indeed to embrace uncertainty and imperfection. — Arianna Huffington

I am Grateful For:

breakfast   lunch   dinner   snacks   exercise

got dressed and ready for the day

30 min. mommy time	personal/spiritual development	went outside
connected with spouse	talked to a friend	asked for help

Feelings, sweet moments, and other notes:

Friday

After all, tomorrow is another day.
- Scarlett O'Hara, Gone with the Wind

I am Grateful For:

breakfast   lunch   dinner   snacks   exercise

~~~~~~~~~~~~~~~~~~~~~~~~~~~~~~~~~

got dressed and ready for the day

30 min. mommy time	personal/spiritual development	went outside
connected with spouse	talked to a friend	asked for help

Feelings, sweet moments, and other notes:

Saturday

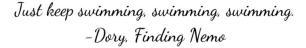

Just keep swimming, swimming, swimming.
–Dory, Finding Nemo

I am Grateful For:

breakfast   lunch   dinner   snacks   exercise

got dressed and ready for the day

30 min. mommy time	personal/spiritual development	went outside
connected with spouse	talked to a friend	asked for help

Feelings, sweet moments, and other notes:

Sunday

I am Grateful For:

breakfast   lunch   dinner   snacks   exercise

~~~~~~

got dressed and ready for the day

| 30 min. mommy time | personal/spiritual development | went outside |
| connected with spouse | talked to a friend | asked for help |

Feelings, sweet moments, and other notes:

Weekly Reflection

My greatest struggle this week was...

I'm proud of myself this week because...

Next week I want to focus on....

I am a great mama.

Monday

The success of every woman should be the inspiration to another. We should raise each other up. — Serena Williams

I am Grateful For:

breakfast   lunch   dinner   snacks   exercise

~~~~~~~~~~~~~~~~~~~~~~~~~~~~~~~~~~~~~~~

got dressed and ready for the day

| 30 min. mommy time | personal/spiritual development | went outside |
| connected with spouse | talked to a friend | asked for help |

Feelings, sweet moments, and other notes:

Tuesday

Be present in all things. Be thankful for all things.
– Maya Angelou

I am Grateful For:

breakfast   lunch   dinner   snacks   exercise

got dressed and ready for the day

| 30 min. mommy time | personal/spiritual development | went outside |
| connected with spouse | talked to a friend | asked for help |

Feelings, sweet moments, and other notes:

Wednesday

I am Grateful For:

breakfast   lunch   dinner   snacks   exercise

got dressed and ready for the day

30 min. mommy time	personal/spiritual development	went outside
connected with spouse	talked to a friend	asked for help

Feelings, sweet moments, and other notes:

Thursday

I now see how owning our story and loving ourselves through that process is the bravest thing that we will ever do.
— Brené Brown

I am Grateful For:

breakfast   lunch   dinner   snacks   exercise

got dressed and ready for the day

| 30 min. mommy time | personal/spiritual development | went outside |
| connected with spouse | talked to a friend | asked for help |

Feelings, sweet moments, and other notes:

Friday

Start children off on the way they should go, and even when they are old they will not turn from it. Proverbs 22:6

I am Grateful For:

breakfast   lunch   dinner   snacks   exercise

~~~~~~~~~~~~~~~~~~~~~~~~~~~~~~~

got dressed and ready for the day

30 min. mommy time	personal/spiritual development	went outside
connected with spouse	talked to a friend	asked for help

Feelings, sweet moments, and other notes:

Saturday

Love is putting someone else's needs before your own.
—Olaf, Frozen

I am Grateful For:

breakfast   lunch   dinner   snacks   exercise

~~~~~~~~~~~~~~~~~~~~~~~~~~

got dressed and ready for the day

| 30 min. mommy time | personal/spiritual development | went outside |
| connected with spouse | talked to a friend | asked for help |

Feelings, sweet moments, and other notes:

Sunday

Self-care is so important. You cannot serve from an empty vessel. –Elanor Brown

I am
Grateful
For:

breakfast   lunch   dinner   snacks   exercise

~~~~~~~~~~~~~~~~~~~~~~~~~~~~~

got dressed and ready for the day

| 30 min. mommy time | personal/spiritual development | went outside |
| connected with spouse | talked to a friend | asked for help |

Feelings, sweet moments, and other notes:

Weekly Reflection

My greatest struggle this week was...

I'm proud of myself this week because...

Next week I want to focus on....

I am a great mama.

Monday

You are fearfully and wonderfully made.
Psalm 139:14

I am Grateful For:

breakfast   lunch   dinner   snacks   exercise

~~~~~~~~~~~~~~~~~~~~~~~~~~~~~~~~~~~~

got dressed and ready for the day

| 30 min. mommy time | personal/spiritual development | went outside |
| connected with spouse | talked to a friend | asked for help |

Feelings, sweet moments, and other notes:

Tuesday

My mission in life is not merely to survive, but to thrive, and do so with some passion, some compassion, some humor, and some style.
—Maya Angelou

I am Grateful For:

breakfast   lunch   dinner   snacks   exercise

~~~~~~~~~~~~~~~~~~~~~~~~~~~~~~~~~~

got dressed and ready for the day

| 30 min. mommy time | personal/spiritual development | went outside |
| connected with spouse | talked to a friend | asked for help |

Feelings, sweet moments, and other notes:

Wednesday

To be honest, I'm just winging it. My life, my eye liner, everything. – Author Unknown

I am Grateful For:

breakfast   lunch   dinner   snacks   exercise

~~~~~~~~~~~~~~~~~~~~~~~~~~~~

got dressed and ready for the day

| 30 min. mommy time | personal/spiritual development | went outside |
| connected with spouse | talked to a friend | asked for help |

Feelings, sweet moments, and other notes:

Thursday

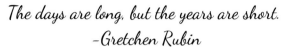

The days are long, but the years are short.
—Gretchen Rubin

I am Grateful For:

breakfast   lunch   dinner   snacks   exercise

got dressed and ready for the day

30 min. mommy time	personal/spiritual development	went outside
connected with spouse	talked to a friend	asked for help

Feelings, sweet moments, and other notes:

Friday

All your kids want is you. Not the fit mom, not the Pinterest mom, not the PTA mom, not every other mom you think you should be. All they want is you, so be the happiest you there was. –Cat & Nat

I am Grateful For:

breakfast   lunch   dinner   snacks   exercise

got dressed and ready for the day

30 min. mommy time	personal/spiritual development	went outside
connected with spouse	talked to a friend	asked for help

Feelings, sweet moments, and other notes:

Saturday

May you be proud of who you are, what you do, and the difference you make. –Author Unknown

I am Grateful For:

breakfast   lunch   dinner   snacks   exercise

~~~~~~~~~~~~~~~~~~~~~~~~~~~~~~~~~~~~~

got dressed and ready for the day

30 min. mommy time	personal/spiritual development	went outside
connected with spouse	talked to a friend	asked for help

Feelings, sweet moments, and other notes:

Sunday

Never underestimate the influence you have on others.
—Laurie Buchanan

I am Grateful For:

breakfast   lunch   dinner   snacks   exercise

~~~~~~~~~~~~~~~~~~~~~~~~~~~~

got dressed and ready for the day

| 30 min. mommy time | personal/spiritual development | went outside |
| connected with spouse | talked to a friend | asked for help |

Feelings, sweet moments, and other notes:

Weekly Reflection

My greatest struggle this week was...

I'm proud of myself this week because...

Next week I want to focus on....

I am a great mama.

Monday

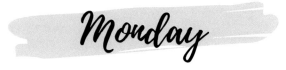

Self-care means giving yourself permission to pause.
—Cecelia Tran

I am Grateful For:

breakfast   lunch   dinner   snacks   exercise

got dressed and ready for the day

| 30 min. mommy time | personal/spiritual development | went outside |
| connected with spouse | talked to a friend | asked for help |

Feelings, sweet moments, and other notes:

Tuesday

You can't simultaneously do it all and do it well. But you can choose to cultivate what matters right where you are. -Lara Casey

I am Grateful For:

breakfast   lunch   dinner   snacks   exercise

~~~~~~

got dressed and ready for the day

| 30 min. mommy time | personal/spiritual development | went outside |
| connected with spouse | talked to a friend | asked for help |

Feelings, sweet moments, and other notes:

Wednesday

Mothering is the gospel lived out as you hold your child's heart in beauty, prayer, and patience. It's not the big decisions, but the little ones, trusting God through it all. -Elizabeth Hawn

I am Grateful For:

breakfast   lunch   dinner   snacks   exercise

got dressed and ready for the day

| 30 min. mommy time | personal/spiritual development | went outside |
| connected with spouse | talked to a friend | asked for help |

Feelings, sweet moments, and other notes:

Thursday

Taking care of myself makes me a better mom because I parent from abundance, rather than lack thereof. -Toni-Ann

I am Grateful For:

breakfast   lunch   dinner   snacks   exercise

~~~~~~~~~~~~~~~~~~~~~~~~~~~~~~~~~~~~~~~

got dressed and ready for the day

| 30 min. mommy time | personal/spiritual development | went outside |
| connected with spouse | talked to a friend | asked for help |

Feelings, sweet moments, and other notes:

Friday

The best and most beautiful things in the world cannot be seen or even touched – they must be felt with the heart.
–Helen Keller

I am Grateful For:

breakfast   lunch   dinner   snacks   exercise

~~~~~~~~~~~~~~~~~~~~~~~~~~~~~~~~~

got dressed and ready for the day

30 min. mommy time	personal/spiritual development	went outside
connected with spouse	talked to a friend	asked for help

Feelings, sweet moments, and other notes:

Saturday

I can't think of any better representation of beauty than someone who is unafraid of herself. -Emma Stone

I am Grateful For:

breakfast   lunch   dinner   snacks   exercise

〰️〰️〰️〰️〰️〰️〰️〰️〰️〰️

got dressed and ready for the day

| 30 min. mommy time | personal/spiritual development | went outside |
| connected with spouse | talked to a friend | asked for help |

Feelings, sweet moments, and other notes:

Sunday

People, even more than things, have to be restored, renewed, revived, reclaimed, and redeemed; never throw out anyone. –Audrey Hepburn

I am Grateful For:

breakfast   lunch   dinner   snacks   exercise

got dressed and ready for the day

| 30 min. mommy time | personal/spiritual development | went outside |
| connected with spouse | talked to a friend | asked for help |

Feelings, sweet moments, and other notes:

Weekly Reflection

My greatest struggle this week was...

I'm proud of myself this week because...

Next week I want to focus on....

I am a great mama.

Monday

Define success on your own terms, achieve it by your own rules, and build a life you're proud to live. —Anne Sweeney

I am Grateful For:

breakfast   lunch   dinner   snacks   exercise

got dressed and ready for the day

30 min. mommy time	personal/spiritual development	went outside
connected with spouse	talked to a friend	asked for help

Feelings, sweet moments, and other notes:

Tuesday

What makes you different or weird, that's your strength.
— Meryl Streep

I am
Grateful
For:

breakfast   lunch   dinner   snacks   exercise

~~~~~~~~~~~~~~~~~~~~~~~~~~~~~~~

got dressed and ready for the day

| 30 min. mommy time | personal/spiritual development | went outside |
| connected with spouse | talked to a friend | asked for help |

Feelings, sweet moments, and other notes:

Tuesday

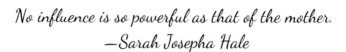

No influence is so powerful as that of the mother.
—Sarah Josepha Hale

I am Grateful For:

breakfast   lunch   dinner   snacks   exercise

got dressed and ready for the day

| 30 min. mommy time | personal/spiritual development | went outside |
| connected with spouse | talked to a friend | asked for help |

Feelings, sweet moments, and other notes:

Wednesday

Live in the moment and make it so beautiful that it will be worth remembering. —Fanny Crosby

I am Grateful For:

breakfast   lunch   dinner   snacks   exercise

~~~~~~~~~~~~~~~~~~~~

got dressed and ready for the day

30 min. mommy time	personal/spiritual development	went outside
connected with spouse	talked to a friend	asked for help

Feelings, sweet moments, and other notes:

Thursday

A baby will make love stronger, days shorter, nights longer, bankroll smaller, home happier, clothes shabbier, the past forgotten, and the future worth living for. —Unknown

I am Grateful For:

breakfast   lunch   dinner   snacks   exercise

got dressed and ready for the day

| 30 min. mommy time | personal/spiritual development | went outside |
| connected with spouse | talked to a friend | asked for help |

Feelings, sweet moments, and other notes:

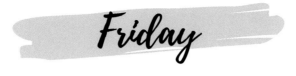

Friday

Empowered women empower women.
-Unknown

I am
Grateful
For:

breakfast   lunch   dinner   snacks   exercise

got dressed and ready for the day

| 30 min.
mommy time | personal/spiritual
development | went
outside |
| connected
with spouse | talked to
a friend | asked
for help |

Feelings, sweet moments, and other notes:

Saturday

There is no place like home.
— Dorothy, The Wizard of Oz

I am Grateful For:

breakfast   lunch   dinner   snacks   exercise

got dressed and ready for the day

30 min. mommy time	personal/spiritual development	went outside
connected with spouse	talked to a friend	asked for help

Feelings, sweet moments, and other notes:

Sunday

You is kind. You is smart. You is important.
— Kathryn Stockett, The Help

I am
Grateful
For:

breakfast   lunch   dinner   snacks   exercise

~~~~~~~~~~~~~~~~~~~~~~~~~~~~

got dressed and ready for the day

30 min. mommy time	personal/spiritual development	went outside
connected with spouse	talked to a friend	asked for help

Feelings, sweet moments, and other notes:

Weekly Reflection

My greatest struggle this week was...

I'm proud of myself this week because...

Next week I want to focus on....

I am a great mama.

Made in the USA
Coppell, TX
05 January 2020

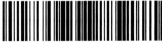

14107556R00062